Jenny

Morgan Stornoway

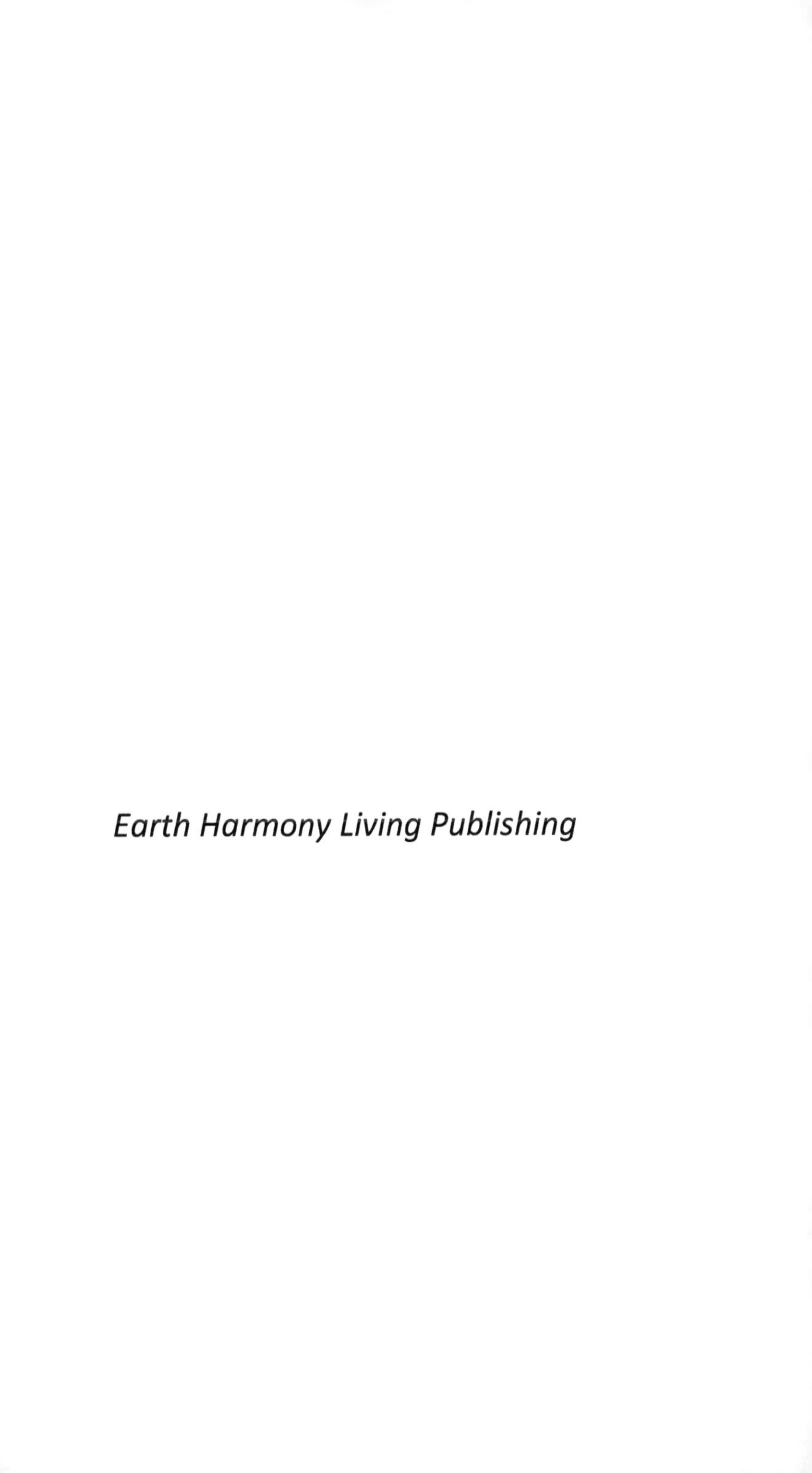

Earth Harmony Living Publishing

Jenny
By Morgan Stornoway
Editor Guenevere MacDonald,
Bethany Rickard-Wood
Published by Earth Harmony Living Publishing

1. Edition, 2021

ISBN 97819904260205

Earth Harmony Living Publishing

Dedicated to anyone who has ever experienced trauma and survived.

To my daughters who love unconditionally

My husband, who has stuck it through

And my editorial team at Earth Harmony Living.

Jenny

As a child, I was called Jennifer, a name I despised with a passion. I wanted to be called something else. At the very least, I wanted to be called Jenny. Jenny, to me, was a nickname that parents used when they really loved you. Jenny was a nickname friends and lovers used as a term of endearment when they really cared about you. Jenny was love and affection. Everyone always called me Jennifer. The only person who called me Jenny was me, and only when I talked to myself.

The name Jenny has always represented a time of sadness for me, but I also connected it to a side of me I do not share with people. Jenny is a part of me, but she is a different person at the same time.

No one knows the inside of my mind, except Jenny and it is a scary, scary place most days. Other days it is perfect. Those are the days I do not want to come back. I want to stay there and be that person forever. Those are the days I am not Jenny. Those are the days when Jenny is gone forever, and it seems she is never coming back. But Jenny always comes back. She haunts me day and night. Jenny is all the most horrible things in life. Jenny means no love…ever, not for me. Jenny means torture and betrayal. Jenny is all things evil and all things wicked. Jenny is the horror of the past, and she steals the future.

Jenny however is also the strong side of me. She can kick some ass when she needs too but more than anything she simply plots, always thinking ahead and what comes next.

For me it's the past that captures my attention.

Linda

My mother was 14 years old when I was born. She once bragged that she was so drunk that night she could not find her way home from the apartment next door. She claimed I was an easy birth and came quickly. Given the amount she had to drink, I don't wonder if I was trying to escape rather than just be born.

She was a heavy drinker, a drug user, and it wouldn't be long after my birth that she became a prostitute of sorts as well.

She was a child of the system—one of seven children with different fathers who were all removed from their mother's care. Three of those children were adopted, three were returned to their mother. Linda had suffered from attachment issues when she was a child and could not form bonds with anyone, so her prospects of adoption were low. All the attempts to adopt her failed. Her mother refused to take her back, so she remained in the system until she was sixteen and she ran away.

At the tender age of thirteen, she discovered she was pregnant; she was in a home for teenaged girls in Nova Scotia at the time. Once her pregnancy was discovered, she was transferred back to the New Brunswick foster care system. Several attempts were made to convince her to terminate the pregnancy. She refused. She always told me that she had done me a great favour with great gusto by holding off the wolves who wanted to destroy me. Someone should have told her early on that she was not a princess, and this was by far not a fairy tale. Had it been one, it would be the worst fairy tale ever written.

After my birth, she attempted to keep me but failed miserably. She just couldn't grasp the concept of providing adequate care. I am told she treated me like a doll and used me to her advantage to get things from others who felt sorry for her. She had very few parental skills, no resources and even less instinct. In retrospect, I do not know why they let her hold on to me for so long. After 22 homes, most of which she was evicted from, constant complaints from neighbours whom she had dropped me off for a "couple of hours," and a pattern of general instability, drugs, and partying, I was removed from her care.

I was placed in foster care, where I experienced the first amount of stability, I had had in my short two years. The foster home was with a young United Pentecostal family with three children. They had a large house and a big backyard with swings and toys. They were experienced foster parents and were extensively used for emergency placements. The older children were used to other kids coming and going and did their part to help with the younger ones. I began to develop a sense of self-confidence in that foster home, but it did not stay that way. Linda took the opportunity to snatch me when the older children accidentally left me outside at lunchtime. From New Brunswick, we headed west to Alberta with police and social services hot on our trail.

Linda sees her act of desperation as saving me from the system. The reality was that she had done me a huge disservice. During her time in Alberta there was no supervision, and no one was checking in on her to see that I was okay and my needs were being met. Most of the abuse I suffered as a child happened in Alberta after I was out of the foster care system and very much at the mercy of my child mother.

Photographs & Memories

My memories always start like photographs that shift and morph into moving pictures. I see my life as an outsider, not as myself. I have always seen things that way from the outside looking in. I often imagine that is what an out-of-body experience must be like. Only mine never seem to join up. I never go back inside my body; I am permanently stuck outside, watching through photographs. I see myself playing or bathing, sleeping or in most cases crying and screaming. I always see the shadows hanging around me while I do these things, like spirits watching over me while I play and go about my life. I recall one early memory of sitting in a tub, and a dark-haired woman is pulling strips of skin off my sunburned arms. I do not cry despite it clearly looking painful, but instead, I play with the toy dishes floating in the tub. I have no idea who the woman is, but she laughs as she peels the skin away. In the background, shadows lurk in the corners, watching.

I remember the day Linda snatched me too. I remember standing in the driveway holding my doll and wondering where everyone went. In the memory, a woman runs up, grabs me, and takes me to the car with a big black man behind the steering wheel. When the vehicle pulls away, a woman comes running behind the car, yelling my name. Which I find ironic because my memory of being in Alberta ends pretty much the same way. Linda runs into the waiting room and yells for the man to take me. He grabs me up and runs out of the building and looks around the corner. The scene looks like New York, and there are police cars. There is a squabble, and I eventually get pulled away and put in the police car. When Linda comes out, she kicks the vehicle as we are driving away. My lasting memory of her from my childhood is her running after the car yelling my name. Ironically it is the only time in my life when I have been called Jenny, and on both occasions, my name is being screamed by desperate women.

I remembered that incident all through my childhood. Years later, when I read the official account in my adoption record, it was described exactly as I had retold the story without ever seeing the file. But what wasn't described explicitly in the file was the dark rooms with strange people and strange noises, the shiny guns, the strange men called uncles or the loud arguments and crashing objects.

Getting me out of that scenario was best. But the group home was just as bad.

The group home was mentioned in the file. It was for older kids, and I remember the tormenting from the older kids., Particularly the kids who tried to steal my doll or the woman who slapped me across the face and shook me when I wouldn't stop screaming over it. Or the fact that I had started to hide from that woman every time I saw her. I hid under beds and in closets, in the cupboards and in the laundry. The woman scared me, and every time I remember her, I see a dark shadow looming behind her.

The photograph I remember the most was the plane ride back east, the dark house, and Ann answering the door. The house was big, quiet, and spooky. I was terrified when I showed up on Patrick and Ann's doorstep. They fussed and fussed over me, but no amount of fussing ever calmed me down. I screamed, and I cried, and I cowered. At some point between that encounter and the actual adoption, they sought professionals to evaluate me. Those professionals advised against the adoption, but Patrick and Ann went ahead and simply dressed me up and posed me for photographs. Photographs with great toys, photographs with expensive clothes, photographs on big vacations. In every picture, they told me to smile. Behind the scenes, the darkness was there, and I was terrified of everything. As far as everyone was concerned, I was an average happy child. I remember differently.

Fear of Everything

Fear of everything best describes my childhood. I was afraid of the wind because it howled my name, the grass because it tried to eat my toes. The trees because they reached out to grab me when I went by. Even the birds followed me and eyed me suspiciously like I was a snack they wanted to carry off. Sand stuck to me and refused to let go and open water was just an invitation to get swallowed up. Photographs from those early years are of two types: smiling happy child looking at the camera and posing as instructed and the child screaming and crying or on the verge of screaming and crying. When I got older and asked Ann for my two photo albums, she refused to give them to me. Eventually, she made a third album that included select photos of me posing and smiling. Every image is posed. Most are birthday photos. They tell a very clear story. To say I was a strange child that had a hard time making friends is an understatement. Every single birthday photograph is clear proof of those issues. Not one photo has the same friends. I never made friends easily, and those friends I had I failed to keep. I never knew one day to the next who would play with me on the playground, and I was constantly bullied because I was an easy target without a group to protect me.

On one occasion, I was backed up to the monkey bars by the school bully Tarah Lynn who demanded that I hand over my gum. I had one piece, and it was in my mouth. The kids encircled me, ready to watch the pounding that was sure to come. I was stuck. I couldn't get away. The teachers stood off in the distance, watching but not intervening. They never got involved until blood was drawn. That day I was either brave or foolish, but for whatever reason, I decided to give her my gum. by spitting it in her face. A voice in my head told me to let her have it. So, without thinking, I did. I spit it right in her eye.

Spitting my gum at her drew laughter and applause from the other kids who started to mock her. She screamed at me but walked away. Promising to get me back. She did the next day, but for that moment, I was feeling bold.

Tormented and teased just about every day, if not every day, I was the last to be picked the first to be picked on, and I was the only kid I knew who was adopted. The school kids knew it, too, since my brother had loudly announced to the whole school that I was such a screw-up that my own parents dumped me in the trash can, and my adoptive parents brought me home like a puppy. I had never felt I belonged before that, but I was the social outcast of the century after that moment.

I was awkward, fearful and no one ever believed me when I spoke. According to my teachers and report cards, my stories of bullying were imaginative, fanciful, and often inappropriate. I was labelled disruptive by more than one teacher for complaining too much.

When I got bold, I did stupid things like cutting a classmate's hair in the bathroom. Her sister kicked my ass the next day. I once decided that I was the greatest scientist in the world, and I would save all the children in Africa by creating super penicillin. For a month, I gathered all the sandwich crusts from every kid in the lunchroom and left them to rot in my desk. I even moved all my school supplies to my book bag and carried them back and forth to school every day, so my mold could grow. When the teacher found out, he was furious and promptly trashed my mold and moved me and my smelly desk to the hall. After school, I rescued my mold and took it home, where I tended it in the playhouse until winter hit and it got destroyed in the snow. I was by all accounts a bizarre kid.

I was a haunted kid too. Everywhere I went, I saw things that other people didn't seem to notice. Shadows, animals, people, and children playing. I heard music and people talking when no one else did. I truly believed I was seeing and hearing ghosts. At one point, I began to carve all their names on the wall in my bedroom. (They told me to do it.) When Ann found out, she and Patrick were furious. Patrick repainted the wall, and they inspected it every night after that. I was rather upset because I felt it was necessary to remember them all, and I needed a way to write them down.

The things I saw and heard were so real to me that when a deluge of water burst through a crack in the foundation wall and flooded my bedroom with ankle-deep ice-cold water, I didn't find it the least bit strange. I just stood there wondering how I was going to explain it. I was worried I would be blamed for it. I was blamed for everything. When Ann came in and saw the water, she said nothing to me. Neither she nor Patrick blamed me, which at the time scared me more than if they had.

Happy Memories

When I try to think back and remember happy memories of my childhood, they are almost nonexistent. I have snapshots in my head of moments that I know should have been happy, but they are not.

Birthdays are simply photographs, and while Christmas feels like it should be more exciting, those memories are also just snapshots in my mind.

I vaguely remember a feeling of Christmas, a sensation that I've tried to recreate over the years. Still, it always ends up leaving me depressed and disappointed.

I believe it's more of an expectation of what it should feel like rather than an actual feeling associated with a particular memory.

Major events like high school and university graduation, the birth of my first child etc. hold no emotion for me.

My wedding memories are of excitement and relief. Excitement for the day and relief when it was over. The event was marred by family members who made a big stink about attending. By the time the actual day rolled around, we were emotionally exhausted. The memory has been pushed aside in my brain as a result.

My two youngest children were high risk pregnancies with one almost dying in delivery and the other almost dying in utero.

It seems every major event in my life has somehow been sullied and affected by a negative emotion leaving little to no room for any positive aspect to leak through.

So, I hold on to the snapshot memories and a belief in the emotion that “should” be associated with the event.

Not Belonging

From the time I became aware of other kids, I knew I didn't belong. My adoption and the 5 years leading up to it were plagued with drama and trauma. To say I was a badly traumatized child was an understatement. The records showed I had been physically and sexually abused, neglected, and abandoned. I'd moved over 22 times in two years, and I was even abducted from a foster home. All before the age of four. The trauma I experienced was why Ann and Patrick were advised not to adopt me in the first place. They had their chance to walk away from the adoption before it even began, but they chose not to. Most likely, they had dreams of saving the poor orphan, but that is not how it turned out.

I'm sure that if they were given a choice today to go back and make that decision again, they would walk away. I am sure this is the only one where I was adopted in all the parallel universes in the universe. I was a troubled and disturbed child, a horrible and deeply damaged teen, and I grew into a broken adult.

Ann and Patrick were warned early on, and yet they did nothing. Despite making the commitment as adoptive parents and knowing my past trauma and abuse, there was no therapy, counselling, and help for me whatsoever. Just demands that I act normal and excel at something like my siblings did. Pressure, ridicule, disbelief, and unrealistic expectations were all that were offered to me.

I never felt I belonged in that family or anywhere else, so I disappeared into my own little world. I had ghosts I could talk to even if no one believed me. I had special abilities even they couldn't see. I heard things no one heard, and I saw things no one saw. They called me fanciful, imaginative, and sometimes straight-up liar. But it only happened more and more as I got older.

There are large portions of my memory missing because I was unaware of what was going on around me. I remember once driving four hours to visit family and then four hours back. But I don't recall driving the return trip, only turning up at the gate and wondering how I got there.

When I think about the things that torment me the most in life, there are two things—the voices and images in my head and childhood. If I had to correct one, it would be my childhood.

Tormented in my head and in life, neglected for my mental health and rejected by the only people I knew to be parents, my childhood was nothing short of a shitpile. No amount of money, possessions or experiences could make up for the overwhelming feeling of abandonment that radiated from Ann and Patrick. Their total abrupt cut-off in my adult years was the final nail in the coffin. While they still professed to care, they stopped calling and messaging outside of holiday greetings and ignore my children outside of holidays and birthdays. Ann would usually try to buy love with gifts without ever speaking to the children or inquiring about their health or interests. A letter would have gone so much further. A phone call would have meant so much more. But money was easier, especially after I saw the hospital files and their comments to doctors about me.

It was clear they did not care and had stopped doing so many years earlier. Likely very soon after the adoption. The pain of realizing this was as profound and as deep as losing the child who ran off without so much as a goodbye, thanks for the memories. But it hurt more so as they continued to just pop up on holidays.

Had I had the chance, I'd have gone back in time and stopped the adoption. Truth be told I should never have been adopted into that family. I would have seen to it I was adopted into a home with no other children and with adults who were willing and able to repair the damage done in my early childhood. Maybe things would have evolved the way they did.

Doreen

When I was 5, I got into an argument with Ann. During the argument, I yelled that I would rather live with her sister. Her sister Doreen had always been so kind and attentive to me when I visited. I never felt left out around her. Ann did not take too kindly to this and promptly packed all my clothes in my suitcase, which she put out on the front step. She shoved me out the door and pointed up the road, and said, "her house is that way." Ann then slammed the door and locked it leaving me on the front step with a suitcase I couldn't move, no coat and no shoes. I tried frantically to get back inside, but she refused to open the door. So, I stood on the front step, screaming and crying to be let back into the house. I probably would have tried to make it to

Doreen's house had I had shoes and not been told the woods along the side of the road were full of bears.

Ann tossed me out right after lunch, and I stayed on the step crying until Patrick came home for supper and let me into the house. I wanted to live with Doreen more than ever after that, but I didn't dare say anything about it. I was sure that had Patrick not come home and let me in, I would have been eaten by the bears in the woods.

I learned on that day if I didn't do as I was told, I would be thrown out. It scared me so bad that I had constant nightmares. I never forgot that afternoon either. Even as a teenager it was a reminder to never push the limits too far. But at the same time, part of me wanted them to toss me out again. The only problem was I had nowhere to go.

Sleepwalking

As a child, I used to sleepwalk late at night. I'd wander around the house and turn on all the lights and rearrange stuff. I'd run into things as well. One night I walked into my brother's room and ran face-first into the aquarium knocking myself out cold and cracking the aquarium. Everyone was pissed for weeks afterward that I had broken the aquarium, and we'd have to wait to get a new one, by which point the fish would probably die.

Another time I was found in the den rearranging all the books by colour and size. Everyone claims I was sleepwalking, but I vividly remember rearranging the books, the front hall closet, and the food pantry. I even redid Ann's China cabinet and reorganized everyone's shoes. All things that had been annoying me. I remember doing it.. but I don't know how I got there to do it.

I had episodes where I would go all night rearranging things, writing, dancing, or engaging in conversations with myself and my people.

My happiest adventures were drama festivals at the university when I was in junior high and high school. Usually, I had my own room because no one wanted to share it with me. Which was fine by me. As soon as we were released by the teachers, I would make a beeline for the university bookstore, buy new writing materials and sweets and head back to the dorms. I would find a way to play hooky for all the activities except the play I was actually in. I would hide out in my room and spend the weekend writing, dancing, conversing, and pigging out on sweets and junk food. I didn't sleep, and I wasn't tired. It was a blast. Occasionally one of the teachers would show up demanding to know where I had been or telling me to attend a meeting of some sort, but outside of that, I was left alone to my own devices to converse with myself and to write, and I loved it. No siblings, no classmates, no bullies, no Ann and no Patrick. Probably my happiest teen memories. I could have stayed like that forever and not cared.

Skipping

I never really wanted to learn how to skip rope. I never asked to learn, and I had no interest in it. But skipping was popular on the playground, and all the girls brought their ropes to school.

I was delighted to watch from the sidelines and just chat with the girls while they jumped rope. I would turn the rope for the other girls and that was enough for me.

Ann thought differently. She thought I should know how to jump rope and she was determined I would learn. So, every day for a good two hours after school, she pushed me to jump rope.

I was terrible at it. I tripped and fell, tearing up my knees and elbows. That didn't' deter her we simply moved from the driveway to the basement and kept going. Rather than tear up my limbs, I just bruised them on the concrete tiles. I cried and complained, and she pushed harder. I resisted, and she pushed harder.

Finally, I managed to jump rope. Poorly, but I did it. Ann was so happy she bought me two new ropes and excitedly shoved me out the door to school.

I marched off to school and happily took up my position, turning rope for the other girls. My new jump ropes never left my bag. Truth be told I had less desire then ever to skip rope. She had taken all the fun out of it. There wasn't much fun to begin with but what there was had gone with her constant badgering for me to learn.

I never did jump rope at school or at home after that point. I just turned the rope and chatted away.

One day on the playground I heard my name being called. When I looked over to the fence, I saw Ann waving at me. When I ran over, she asked why I was not skipping rope with the other girls. I made a poor excuse about taking turns, but she didn't buy it. She had been watching me the whole recess.

I finally just told her I didn't like jumping rope. She protested, I insisted. It wasn't the first time I had told her I hated jumping rope. I'd been telling her all along. I hated it now more than ever.

She was so upset that she just kept repeating how she had wasted her time, and from then on, I would have to learn things on my own.

I sometimes wonder where the adults were during my childhood. I had never asked to learn to jump rope. In fact, I had protested loudly that I wasn't the least bit interested in it. Yet, I was forced to learn. Ann had pushed and pushed and pushed. I had told her repeatedly no, but she pushed anyway. And here we were standing at the playground fence with her having a meltdown about her wasted time and efforts like a sulking child. It made no difference to me. I never skipped rope after that.

Years later, she sent two jump ropes to my kids… one taught herself the other just set it aside with zero interest. I said nothing. But I remembered.

My people

My people are people no one else can see. They are people I see wherever I go. Some I see only once; some a few times others have stayed with me over the years. I’ve given names to some of my people it makes it easier to talk to them. Some have names already, and they tell me so. My people tell me stories. They tell me what to do and how to talk. Some are kind, and some are cruel. Some I wish would go away, and others I wish would come back. I wish Mary would come back. She was always around when I was a child and when I was in high school. One day I ended up in the hospital. When I got out, she was gone. Deidre too. In their place was the narrator. He is not my people. He is annoying as fuck. I don’t need my life narrated; I know how sad and pathetic it is already. I wish the narrator would go, but Alex and Harry, I hope, will stay forever.

Demons

Today I was called fat; today, I was called a slut and a whore. Not by strangers, not by people I know but by my demons. They call me horrible names. They tell me I am ugly, useless, and worthless. They tell me no one loves me or cares whether I live or die. They taunt me and ridicule me telling me to throw myself down the stairs and to cut myself open and bleed all over. My demons tell me no one would care, and no one would notice. Most days, I know this is not true. My husband and children would be devastated. My demons still tell me they hate me, and I am a horrible wife and mother. Most days, I can fight this. some days, I believe it.

The Hum

There is a hum in my head. A steady nonstop hum. It is the hum of voices. Hundreds of voices all talking to each other. I cannot decipher what they say, but they say it anyway. Like all day, they talk. All night they talk when I am tired. They shout. When I am upset or stressed, they scream. They talk separately; they scream separately, not one voice but hundreds just screaming and sometimes crying, moaning, laughing at each other and at me. I don't know. Sometimes they are quiet, and a slight hum in the background is just loud enough to know they are there. Sometimes it's so loud that I cover my ears, but it does no good because there inside my head. The hum continues. The hum never stops. Even when the narrator speaks and when the demons yell. When my people talk or my soul screams and cries, the hum never stops.

No one Noticed, and No one cared.

I once got lost in the woods. My grandparents lived a good 30 minutes from our house. I left home one day with just a backpack, determined that I was leaving, and I would find myself a proper home. I walked out the door at 730am and didn't look back. I had no idea where to go, so I headed for my grandparent's house and the trails near it. At some point, I got confused and wandered off the path I was familiar with. I spent the better part of the day frantically running in circles, believing I was being chased by shadow people trying to find my way out of the woods. I was terrified, I was hungry, and I was on my own in the woods. Eventually, I managed to get through the woods to the road. I followed it for some time before I discovered I was clear across town by the old Morrissey bridge. A good two-hour walk from my house. When I eventually made it home and walked in the door, I got growled at for not being home before twilight. I had been gone for over 12 hours, and no one had cared. I was 11 years old, and I was convinced beyond all doubt that I well and truly didn’t belong.

Dancing by myself

I would often spend hours in my room talking to Mary and Deidre and other people who would show up. I would spend hours lost in conversation with them and with myself. I'd often lose myself in these conversations, forgetting homework, chores, and meals. I have forgotten all their names over the years, but each one brought something new to my life and would tell me how to do things, where to go, and how to react to different situations. With each new person, I would find myself researching new topics and new experiences and historical accounts. I became knowledgeable on various subjects, but I never excelled at any. Truth be told, I managed to make it through high school only because of this. Benjamin was the lawyer, and because of him, I got an

A in legal studies, but Clarissa barely managed to help me pass my French immersion classes. No one could help me with math and chemistry, and I finally passed those on the second try.

I remember happy times spent immersed in scenarios with these people. But not all of them were kind, and not all of them were visible. The ones that didn't show themselves were the worst. They got nastier the older I got. They told me horrid things and encouraged me to do things that almost always got me in trouble or scared me to death and made me look like an idiot.

I was trying so hard to fit in at school the whole time, but still, I couldn't manage to keep the same friends. When I was lost for something to do or say, I almost always listened to what was in my head. Which clearly seemed to be weirdly inappropriate or off-topic 99 percent of the time.

This always leads to more teasing, fighting alienation or trouble with grown-ups. I could never figure out how or why I was doing things so wrong. Everyone said to listen to your heart, your conscience, or your gut. So I listened to what the voices in my head said. And I just kept getting into trouble, so I kept our conversations to us. Long hours in my room pacing, walking in circles talking just my people and me. I didn't need friends at that point I had plenty of private ones that were always there. I didn't need anymore bullies either I had plenty of those as well.

The Narrator

If you have ever watched a nature show narrated by David Attenborough, then you know what it sounds like in my head. For some reason, David Attenborough narrates my life. Where I go, every detail, what I do, who I talk to, and even what I think. He is a constant pain in the ass; only he’s in my head. Occasionally my demons mock him, so it sounds like an echo in my head. Sometimes one, sometimes two, sometimes more. It's never quiet.

The Puddle

I turned around in my room one day, and there was a massive black puddle on the floor. Every time I moved, it rippled. It looked thick like mud but smelled foul, like garbage and sewer waste. It covered the floor from one end of the room to the other. I looked over the edge, and the liquid would fall away, leaving a deep hole. I couldn't make out a bottom it just seemed to go on forever, one massive hole in my floor. It scared me. It felt like it wanted to consume me. My heart raced, my hands shook, and I felt cold. So cold, like I was outside in the snow. Everything about it terrified me. In my head, a voice told me it would eat me and sear the flesh off my bones at the same time. That only my skeleton would be left if I went near it. And after a while, my bones would be gone too. No one would find me, and no one would save me. I'd be lost forever, gobbled up by this hideous pit.

I couldn't move. I couldn't speak. I wanted to yell out for someone to come and rescue me, but I couldn't form the words. I couldn't say anything, let alone yell for help. I was stuck in the corner with no way out, and this horrible satanic puddle coming closer and closer. I jumped on my bed but doing so only made it move faster. It started to eat away at the legs of the bed and the dresser. There was no escaping it.

At some point, I started to cry, but it felt like my tears were burning my face. Somewhere I could hear my name being called. I tried to answer but felt as though I was choking trying to get the words out. That was the point when Ann showed up at the door. She called me saying dinner was ready and they were waiting on me. I tried to tell her about the puddle, but the words would not come out correctly. She growled at me for wasting time and told me to come. I tried to warn her again, but she failed to listen. She marched across the room, her feet sinking deeper in the puddle as she came towards me. The puddle hissed and spewed with smoke rising from her legs which were melting before my eyes. I tried to yell for help but felt as though hands were closing around my throat. She reached out and grabbed hold of my hand and pulled. She said everyone is waiting. I pulled back in fear and tried to tell her the danger we were in. She grabbed my other hand and pulled come on, she said. I resisted. I could smell a putrid smell in the room and was painfully aware of the sound of something sizzling. I was sure it was her legs. Yet, she showed no sign of discomfort or pain. She reached out and grabbed both my hands this time and told me to come. I resisted, but being a child, it was a futile effort on my part to getaway. I was being pulled off the bed toward the enormous flesh-eating pit. The room began to spin, my heart raced even more and slowly, I began to lose sensation in my arms and feet. I felt so cold. I cried and tried to break free. In my mind, I was running, but I was very much held in place by my fear. Seldom have I felt such fear as when the other world rears its head. No human has ever caused me such anxiety. No animals have ever threatened my existence the way this did. It wasn't just my body I needed to protect; I felt it was my soul. I was sure that whatever that puddle was, there was no going to heaven if it got a hold of me

So, I kicked, and I cried and screamed. Ann pulled me forward. I pulled back in an endless tug of war. Eventually, she succeeded in pulling me off the bed. I have a vivid recollection of falling toward that black abyss. Then being cold and wet. Lying on the floor in the doorway of my room Ann and Patrick looking at me with horror and disgust. I had clearly pissed them off again, but I didn't care. I could breathe again, and I was away from the man-eating puddle.

The Brother

Growing up, I had five siblings: four brothers (adoptive) and one sister (adoptive). I found out much later, I also had three half-brothers. All of them had biological siblings except for Jonathan, who didn't care one way or another. He had been adopted when he was a newborn, so Jeremy and Don were his brothers biological or otherwise didn't matter.

The worst sibling by far was Jeremy. He was selfish, bossy cruel and violent. He would take every chance he had to threaten me, slap me or take my toys. On one occasion, he came into my room and grabbed my ear and pulled. I had just gotten my ears pierced, and he split the lobe drawing blood. He was never punished for his antics, and often, the tables would be turned around, and I would be blamed for the ruckus and punished.

Jeremy constantly accused me of doing things I didn't do even when I was too small to do them. I took the blame for a good deal of his rotten behaviour. His favourite thing in the world was to tell me no one loved me and no one wanted me. My demons remind me of Jeremy and his wicked ways.

I have a photo of us on the PEI ferry during summer vacation. In the photo, everyone is looking at the camera, smiling except for me. I'm watching Jeremy and clutching a doll to my chest. I had just gotten that doll before we boarded the boat, and he threatened to throw it overboard and then to push me in. He was kind enough to tell me there were sharks in the water too. Jeremy was and still is a horrible, hateful creature of Satan.

Friends are like Diamonds, Precious and rare

I had one friend in junior high and high school that kind of stuck it out with me. We were close in junior high. But in high school, we started to go our separate ways more often. We fought a lot. I usually started it. I was always paranoid that she would go off and be someone else's best friend that I often drove her mad. In the end, she did become someone else's best friend, and I was left with no one. Years later, we reconnected online, but it wasn't the same anymore. Too many years had passed to many things had happened for us to be as close as we had been back in junior high. In truth, I have no one but my husband. I know people that I consider friends but no one to hang out with or chat with every day. No one that I could call in a crisis without feeling I was disturbing them. Only my husband. No, not even family, just him. And there are things I can't even tell him in a crisis that I don't feel would be an inconvenience to him. I have no one in that regard. My deepest, most personal thoughts and feelings are only shared with people I wish really existed.

Sex

My first adventures with sex occurred when I was 14. I was infatuated with a boy named Adam. He was oddly enough also interested in my weird self. I had this idea in my head that I needed to give myself to him. I never did. Ann got wind of what was going on and put a kabosh on it real fast. Not that, that was a bad thing overall. But she decided the best way to put an end to my "ideas" was to park me at the dining room table every night and make me copy over an entire 1970's medical encyclopedia on reproduction, birth and families. The words meant nothing to me as I was lost in my head within five minutes and copied the pages on autopilot without ever absorbing them. She would have been better off explaining the subject to me, but beyond our very awkward discussion on monthly cycles, sex was never discussed in any form. I knew nothing.

All her efforts did was stall me for a few more months, by which time I was convinced I had to do it to save my soul from leaving me. It sounds so strange now, but at the time, I was convinced that if I didn't have life put back in, all my soul would bleed out.

So determined to see it through, I lost my virginity at 15 and became a mother at 19.

For the better part of my first pregnancy, there was a lot of anger, especially on Patrick's part. He didn't speak to me for almost three years. If I was in his house and in his way, he would put his hands on my shoulders and physically move me out of the way. If I had the information he needed, he would rather leave the room without hearing it rather than hear it from me.

For my part, I was relieved my soul was safe and had been secured for a reasonable period. My concern was the delivery, but not because I was afraid of the pain involved, although I told people I was. I was more concerned that my soul would bleed out in the delivery. I was relieved when it was over, and I was still me. At least in some small way, I wasn't entirely sure the child hadn't claimed some. My head told me she had, so when the social worker came to see if I had decided on adoption, I flat out refused and sent her away. Part of me wanted to be a mother—a small part. Part of me wanted to piss off Patrick for the way he had treated me all those years. But mostly, I wanted to keep hold of all my parts, even the one that had departed from me. Despite everything, I still made sure that I never lost my soul. For years I sought out regular partners to replenish my life force, so my soul stayed put. But it wasn't until I married that I allowed myself to become pregnant again.

Bugs on the wall

I'm not afraid of bugs usually. I simply kill them or move away from them. Spiders don't scare me, but I'm not their biggest fan either. It has taken me a long time to get to that point. But when they are together in groups and take over, it's more than a bit much.

I remember being in my room and having dozed off on the bed when a voice screamed in my ear to wake up. I opened my eyes to see something black moving across the ceiling above me. At first, it just seemed like a black mass, but then I realized it was spiders. Hundreds of spiders across the ceiling, the walls and the bed. They started to crawl up my legs over my body and up to my face. I screamed and screamed, which woke up everyone in the house. Ann came running and started to shake me when I wouldn't stop screaming.

But I couldn't stop. I felt each little leg crawling along my skin up, my legs across my arms and even in my mouth crawling across my tongue. I tried to spit them out and scream at the same time. I ended up hyperventilating. Ann was shaking me violently at this point while I waved my arms frantically, trying to shake off the bugs. Finally, Patrick came into the room and drug me off the bed and out the door. Yelling and hollering, they dropped me in the tub and turned on the cold shower. I was soaked, clothes and all. I'd have screamed bloody murder over the ice-cold water, except spiders don't like cold water, and these ones seemed to scatter.

Once I had calmed down enough to explain that my room was full of spiders, I was ordered to return to bed. Patrick and Ann insisted there was nothing in my room, but I refused. I could see the spiders on the wall and the ceiling from the hallway. They told me to return to bed or stand in the hall all night. I refused to go to bed. I stood outside the room dripping wet shivering for the better part of the night when Patrick came back out and ordered me into my room. So I stood just inside the doorway with my back to the side portion of the door. In the morning, I woke up sitting against the end of the door. My back was torn apart from sliding down the door and against the locking mechanism when I fell asleep standing up.

Ann and Patrick grounded me for being disruptive and keeping everyone up half the night. They took my library card and took the book I was reading, Fahrenheit 451 by Ray Bradbury. Everyone knows a book about burning books gives you" nightmares" about spiders.

No Filter

My mouth got me in so much trouble growing up. Either shit would come out unfiltered, or it would come out at the wrong time and place. I used to say things that had nothing to do with what was going on or even wholly inappropriate. Most should have just been left unsaid. Often, I was just as surprised as other people at that came out of my mouth. I had no filter then, and I have no filter now. So, I try to stay quiet, but it doesn't work. Often, I feel I'm watching myself saying things and thinking that girl is nuts. Then I realize that girl is me and I've said something stupid again. Better to keep my mouth shut.

As a teenager, I often said very wrong things and got into trouble with teachers, Patrick and Ann, activity coordinators. Even the confessional priest admonished me for my inappropriate mouth. It wasn't that I intentionally said these things. I don't try to piss people off with my mouth, but it happens non the less. Not only is there no filter, but there is also no stop sign. Things come out of my mouth before I can stop them. I realize how they don't mesh with the situation, but only after people have reacted to what I have said.

Shadow Spider Man

When dinner is served, you sit quietly in your assigned seat and eat everything on your plate. You chew quietly, you say nothing unless you are addressed, and you remember to excuse yourself when you finish. At least you ask to be excused, and you wait for permission to leave. But supper time is seldom without issue. If you chew too loudly, you will be sent off. If you don't eat your hot soup, you will be threatened. If you attempt to eat your hot soup but use your teeth to remove the hot soup ingredients from the spoon, you will be struck up the side of the head. It's simply how it's done.

Should you wish for sweets that someone else has fun will be made at your expense in the form of a piece of raw onion. Whoever thought it was a great practical joke to give a four-year-old raw onion instead of chocolate must be on the sadistic side. But then who punches a six-year-old in the head for eating hot soup when ordered to do so. Ann and Patrick, that's who.

Perhaps the worse meal I ever had was when I was 15 years old. A year after the puddle incident and I was no closer to ridding myself of my demons.

Sitting at the dinner table could be such torture at times, and that meal was no different. I remember the voices telling me that they were coming. I didn't know who they were, but when unseen voices scream that someone is coming to get you, you take notice.

My palms were sweaty, and my fork kept slipping out of my hand. It did not go unnoticed by Ann and Patrick. They issued their usual threat of bed without supper, grounding, or loss of privileges. I was all for going to bed without supper but was grounded instead after "intentionally" dropping my fork a fourth time. My fear was growing the longer I sat there. In my head, the voices kept warning me that they were coming.

After what seemed like an eternity, I finally managed to choke out a request to be excused, which Ann and Patrick quickly shot down. There was no getting away. I kept my eyes down and muttered that I wasn't feeling well, but that went ignored. I tried to focus on my breathing which was coming fast and shallow, but it did no good. I started to feel light-headed, and just when I thought I was going to fall out of my chair, I caught a glimpse of something out of the corner of my eye. It moved so fast. First, I wasn't sure I had actually seen something. But then it passed again slower this time. I froze in place, feeling as though the air had been sucked out of my lungs. In my head, the voices raged and screamed. In front of me, I stared at the dark shadow that loomed behind Jonathan. A dark shape of a person with no discernable face but the look of pure evil. The shadow stood still staring me down before it turned and started crawling up the wall and across the ceiling like a spiderman. My last recollection of that dinner was grabbing my chest in a vain attempt to breathe. This horrid shape slowly descended on me from the ceiling.

Later that night, I woke up to that same creature standing at the end of my bed. It was my first experience with the shadow people. Still, after so many other terrifying experiences, I was determined not to experience it again.

The next day with the voices raging in my ears, I took several handfuls of pills and tried to end my life.

Hospital at 15

My hospital experience wasn't much better than my home experience. I was put in a room by myself that I was sure was haunted. A woman sat in the chair starring at me. Nurses came and went and paid no attention to her whatsoever. When I inquired as to who she was, they seemed puzzled. Finally, when I began to cry because of her menacing stares and finger-pointing, a nurse calmly held my hand and informed me she wasn't there.

This woman was one of several I saw over the years. Another dark-haired woman named Mary had visited me frequently in our house. I was certain she was a lost soul. Everyone told me there was no such thing. Deirdre was another girl who visited me. She would stand in the corner and sing quietly. I could never make out the words, but the songs were soft and sad and oddly comforting.

The woman in the hospital room was not like Mary or Deidre, who just watched me and let me talk to them. This woman was mean and threatening. She made horrid gestures, and my head told me she would kill me in my sleep. So, I didn't sleep. I was relieved when I was transferred to another hospital in another city. I have no recollection of how I got there. I'm pretty sure they drugged me. They put me in a small room by myself with a woman who sat at the door watching me with a clipboard. I don't know how long I was in that room, but it seemed like weeks. I wasn't alone, although they kept telling me I was. The shadow people were now a constant thing. They lurked in every corner and at the end of every bed. I couldn't escape them in the room, and the staff wouldn't let me leave the room except to be escorted to the bathroom.

Beyond all possible belief, someone had left me with a glass juice bottle, and after finishing it, I threw it at the shadow at the end of my bed. The explosion of glass brought all the staff running. Probably a good thing they did because I was seriously eyeing that glass. I never got the chance to get near it. I was injected and restrained immediately. No one even asked why I had thrown it. The sight of the needle and the restraints sent me into a screaming fit of rage. I was tired of being held captive and being threatened constantly. Only the shot calmed me down, and from that point on, I was injected regularly. I spent the rest of my time in that room, lying on the bed staring at the wall. I didn't dare look anywhere else, and the medication slowed everything to a crawl around me. When I did look around, the room was crawling with spiders and shadows. So, I stared at the wall until finally, they informed me they were moving me to another room.

The new room came with the freedom to roam the halls and visit the common room. It gave me a reprieve of sorts from the staff but not from the voices in my head or the shadows in the corners. They told me the medicine would stop that, but it didn't, and they insisted that I must be exaggerating.

On several occasions, I broke and threw myself on the floor, screaming and crying. I have vague memories of people standing over me trying to grab my hands and feet. I remember them whispering in the doorway after putting me back in the first room all over again. I remember the shadows and feeling cold all the time—the sensation of spiders crawling on me and the smell of smoke. But mostly, I remember being in a fog and not being able to get away. They kept telling me I had an illness. I told them repeatedly I wasn't sick; I was haunted.

Hooky

I used to play hooky from school while at school. No one seemed to notice my absences, nor did they care. They never let on if Patrick and Ann knew, so I'm pretty sure they had no idea.

I had found a way to get in and out of various storage areas in the schools' theatre. The theatre was also the community theatre. It seated several hundred people, had a fly gallery and a catwalk. There were multiple dressing rooms, storage areas and staging areas not used by students except during large productions twice a year. Most community events took place on weekends and over the summer months. The rest of the time, these areas sat undisturbed. That is until I found a way to break in.

Some days I would sit up on the catwalk and watch the theatre classes or the band practices. Other days I headed for my favourite spot, the huge basement storage area. It was massive, secure from trespassers and soundproof. Anyone coming in that didn't know the trick to the doors had to use a key, and the doors made a lot of noise, so I had more than enough warning to hide, not that I did very often. It was rare that anyone went down there. It was mostly used for storing old textbooks and theatre props.

It was the perfect place to deal with my demons, talk to my people and get away from prying eyes and judgemental looks. I could pace and talk, sing and rock as needed. If I argued with them, no one would hear me but them and myself. I spent a good deal of time in those rooms, and no one knew about it.

On one occasion, I brought my friend when we were on speaking terms. She liked it there but was nervous about being caught, so she never came back with me. On another occasion, I brought my boyfriend. I lost my virginity that day. Ann would have been furious if she thought I was whoring about in the school basement. She need not have worried. I never took him back there, and neither one of them knew how to manipulate the locks to get in if I wasn't there to open them.

That area was my sacred space, and aside from those two occasions, I never brought anyone down there. This made it so much easier to deal with my demons. During the summer months, I took to the woods. I found a clearing deep in the woods where no one else went. I would spend hours dealing with demons, letting my guard down while simultaneously trying to keep everything held in place and controlled. I was sure if Ann and Patrick knew, they would lock me up and throw away the key for sure.

I was not a normal kid, and they didn't care for that at all. It wasn't how things were done in our family. As far as the rest of the world was concerned, we were a perfectly normal, happy family. We pretended to be exactly that, and everyone outside our home pretended to believe it.

Free the Demons

I once had a teacher who was a real prick. He fancied himself one of the popular kids and coddled the cliques and the jocks. He gave them extra marks, the best theatre roles, and every opportunity for advancement.

Despite my good marks in English and Drama, he refused to write a letter of recommendation. He seemed to have a personal vendetta against me. For years I envisioned him hanging by the neck from a tree. My demons told me it was a fine idea, and I should encourage him. I literally danced when he did kill himself years later—one less miserable bully to call me down and ridicule me in front of others.

I wasn't so fortunate about some of the other teachers who had picked on me and tormented me through the years. Perhaps it's in poor taste, but I cried tears of joy when I found out he had died.

If I had the chance, I would unleash my demons on every person who ever treated me poorly I would hope and pray that my demons would scream and holler, belittle and degrade them the way they do me. I would pray that they would bring them to the brink of suicide, slowly pushing them to the very edge then allowing them to step back before pushing them out again. I would hope that they would wake in the night to bone-chilling screams and find the shadowy outline of a person at the end of their bed watching them. That they would be driven to insanity by a thousand voices talking, suffer the fatigue and paranoia of someone watching and commenting on their every move. Face the mirror as unseen voices tell them how fat and worthless, they are. And once, they took that step to stand on the edge. I'd like to be there to give them that one final shove off the edge.

Insomnia

Nighttime is a restless time for me. I don’t sleep long, and I don’t sleep well. My nights are plagued with insomnia, night terrors, anxiety, and sleep paralysis. I see shadows lurking in the corners all night long. Shapeless people with eyes staring at me slink about the room edging closer every time I close my eyes. I dream horrid dreams of death and murder. When I wake from these nightmares, I cannot move or speak or stop what is transpiring. Many nights my husband has woken to my moaning. At the same time, I desperately try to yell at the horrible creatures in my nightmares.

I've tried every drug imaginable to help me sleep, and none have worked. I’ve tried relaxation techniques, reading, meditating and exercise. I’ve cut the caffeine, the evening meal and the tv before bed. But nothing stops them. Not even the antipsychotics, which in conjunction with my lack of sleep, just make me fat. Nothing helps the sleep issues, and when sleep does come, it's terrifying.

I do not exist

I am not who I think I am. I am not who they think I am. No one knows who I am. The real me does not exist in this world. The real me is somewhere else all the time. Only my shadow is here.

I’m Special

When I was younger, I thought I was special, that I had a gift and could see things others couldn't. Or that I somehow could communicate with the dead. I’m still not entirely sure it's not true.

No one told me that my biological mother was schizophrenic. I found that out after I was diagnosed with schizoaffective disorder. No one told me that at 4 years old, psychologists recommended I be institutionalized. No one told me that at 15, I had been diagnosed with schizophrenia, and no one made any effort to do anything about it.

Another doctor thought I was too young for a diagnosis, Patrick and Ann thought I was a problem child. They all agreed not to tell me and not to tell anyone outside the family. Patrick and Ann didn't even tell their parents. No one knew. They all just thought I was trouble and abnormal. A kid prone to get themselves into trouble whenever it crossed my path.

In high school, I got suspended over a key. Something I still think was over the top ridiculous, but it happened regardless. Ann and Patrick, oddly enough, must have felt the same because rather than make a big stink about it, they took me to the Moncton to go shopping. Truth be told, I was completely befuddled about the situation and had no idea what I had done wrong. Perhaps it was the one and only time where Patrick and Ann backed me up, but then they could have just been cushioning the bigger blow coming down the line, their decision to make me miss my prom. I missed the prom the parties and barely made it to my graduation because they and my brother had decided the day after prom was a great time for him to get married in Ontario. I often wonder why my graduation wasn't considered during the wedding planning and if they were so pissed at me that making me miss such a momentous event was worth it. I never forgot that, and I'm still bitter over it to this day.

Growing Pains

Somewhere in my early teens, I started to develop pains in my legs. I complained about it frequently but was told it was nothing more than growing pains. The pains only worsened with age, and after years of torment, it was finally diagnosed as fibromyalgia. When I finally had a name for it, I told Ann. She poo-pooed the idea that there was legitimately something wrong with me. YEARS LATER, when I was in a car wreck that destroyed my back and balance, she poo-pooed it again, stating it wasn't nearly as bad as I let on.

This was par for the course for her as she never seemed to take anything I said seriously. Despite a diagnosis and prescription for an inhaler, she refused to believe I had asthma, and the pneumonia that I suffered from in 9th grade that lasted for months wasn't "that bad," according to her. So imagine my surprise when she neither denied nor downplayed my diagnosis of schizoaffective disorder.

In fact, her reaction was more that of a person who had known all along. As it turned out, they did know Schizophrenia was the diagnosis I was given after my hospitalization at 15. Something I wasn't treated for or told about. I only found out about the diagnosis after my final diagnosis over 20 years later. In the interim, I have been diagnosed with OCD, clinically depressed, manic depressive (bipolar) and eventually schizoaffective Bipolar type.

The diagnosis validated all my experience with hearing and seeing things no one else could. On the one hand, it proved I hadn't been lying. But on the other hand, it proved that there was absolutely nothing special about me once and for all. My one unique ability turned out to be a mental illness, not a sixth sense ability to see and talk to the dead. The realization that I had been diagnosed but untreated was the nail in the coffin for me as far as Patrick and Ann were concerned. I shut down. I no longer needed nor wanted their love or their approval because I knew beyond all doubt that they had neither to give me.

Who am I

I don’t know who I am most days. Most days, I wake up confused, feeling like I am out of my body. That the body I have does not belong to me. I feel that the life I have does not belong to me. I feel displaced and disoriented. I must convince myself that it’s right even when I don’t want it to be right. I have to ground myself when I know it’s right even though I don't want to. I want to retreat into my mind and be someone else somewhere else. Then I have to bring myself back, again and again, realizing I’m not who I thought I was. I didn’t do what I thought I did, not knowing most of the time what is real and what isn’t. Changing between lives and stories, sounds, and sights, nothing I see or hear is believed I don’t even know if this is real.

Meeting my Mother

I met my biological mother when I was 20 years old. Unfortunately, she did little to impress me. Although she was kind, she was flighty, inconsistent, and prone to quick-changing moods. I had always hoped to meet her again one day and prove all the records and reports about her wrong. But it was clear that as she got older, her condition had gotten worse.

She was insistent that there had been a conspiracy between Ann and her social worker to take me away from her. She was adamant that they had plotted together against her since the day I was born. I'm not a genius by any stretch of the imagination; I struggle with simple math most days, but it didn't take much to see that adoption is a much bigger process than two conspiring women. Especially when a mother's rights have to be taken away.

The reality was she simply couldn’t care for me. Her mental health was bad enough before I was born. She claimed she had been abused in foster homes. She could not form attachments to people and had no family relations to help her. She cared more for herself than me and left me in conditions that were strife with abuse and neglect. I was exposed to drugs, alcohol, weapons, and violence before the age of 4.

So bad was that exposure that I spent years hiding my sibling's toy guns whenever I had the chance. I screamed at everything, and you couldn’t convince me that uncles did not share the bed with mommies. To this day, I have an intense and rather depraved view of sex that can only be explained by the prior abuse.

Yet for all her faults, Linda was open and honest, and she believed what she believed, and she had honestly tried her hardest to hold on to me. The best efforts of a child but effort, nonetheless.

One could not say the same for Patrick and Ann. They couldn't be more opposite in all things. Patrick and Ann had education, good careers, and knowledge of my background. They knew of the abuse and the extent that it had affected me. They had sought counsel and psychiatric evaluations of me before my adoption. Yet, despite being warned against it, they went through with the adoption anyway.

Now common sense will dictate that if you take in a child with these issues, you make an effort to correct the damage done for everyone's sake. No, they didn't do that. They carried on as though nothing had ever happened, and the simple act of caring for me could fix everything. In all honesty, they should never have been allowed to adopt me. They had three other children, and within two years of my adoption, they took in two more special needs kids. I was left to my nightmares and my demons as priorities were determined by who yelled the loudest or achieved the most.

They once complained that I had deviant and attention-seeking behaviour. Yes, I did. I needed help. I begged for help the only way I knew how, and they ignored it. Only when I forced their hand by trying to kill myself did they do anything about it. And boy did the truth come out then. I didn't find out what they said until years later, but it proved what I had felt all along when the files were released. I was the one purchase they made that they couldn't return. They were unhappy from my arrival. They blamed all the discord in the home on me as well as any problems in their marriage. That's a lot to blame a little kid for. Especially one you knew was damaged, to begin with. But despite it all and despite a diagnosis and recommendation, they ignored it all, stopped treatment and pretended that we were a perfectly normal family. So, first chance they got to cut ties with me, they did.

Linda might have had her faults. She never knew any better, and no one took the time to help her either, but of the two "mothers," one is as bad as the other on the surface. Underneath, Linda can claim honest ignorance for the abuse she put me through, but Ann knew better and did nothing, which is its own form of abuse.

Ann

My memories of her are yelling, screaming, and fighting. I remember endless spankings, groundings, and chores. I don't remember hugs or any form of closeness. Her idea of fixing problems was to spend money. There was never any understanding or compassion when I told her what I was experiencing. I was to her a liar, a child who exaggerated. I couldn't be trusted in any way. There was no sympathy; there was no help.

When the shadows struck and terrorized me, I was sent back to bed with threats of endless punishments. Things I saw were nightmares, stories or lies. My pleas for help were ignored.

Only when I tried to take my own life was anything taken seriously. But even then, recommended therapy was not done, medication was stopped, and I was expected to carry on like a normal child filling the footsteps of my overachieving siblings.

I tried. I was enrolled in guides, but they never participated in activities. I was often forgotten at meetings and left to walk home alone in the cold and dark. I played ringette, but they never came to practices or games even though we lived across the street from the arena. Figure skating was the same, and they missed all my big competitions. When I cried and complained, they simply took me out of the sport or activity. The same thing happened with track and field, cross country running, tennis and field hockey.

Something I was never relieved of was the household chores or babysitting my younger siblings. Ann made it clear that my role as a future mother and wife warranted learning how to run a household. This was not entirely untrue, but the chores in the household were disproportionally unequal in distribution. Yet if I protested, the hammer fell. So, I spend many hours each week lost in my head on autopilot, washing dishes, dusting, scrubbing bathrooms and sitting in the playroom with my younger siblings or folding laundry. In my head, I wasn’t even there I was lost in conversations with other people, lost in scenes that took me far away from Ann and her demands, her yelling, and her endless punishments.

Patrick was another story. He hated me. I knew that from the beginning. There was no closeness with him whatsoever. He avoided conversations and activities with me. Often, he forgot to pick me up from events. While he attended practices and tournaments for my sibling's activities, he never attended my sporting events. Ever. Not once. He often came down heavy on me, never listened to anything I said with any amount of compassion or care. The only times I ever heard him swear were about me or at me.

I grew up being told I was special because I was adopted and chosen; it became clear I was not there by their choice. I was what was available at the time, and there were no substitutions, exchanges, or refunds. While Ann may have initially thought that she could somehow fix me, Patrick held no such beliefs. He was miserable since my arrival and said as much to my doctors when I was hospitalized.

Their comments regarding how they felt about me were recorded in the file for posterity. A file I saw later in life confirming everything I thought as a child and everything my head told me. I was cared for, but I wasn't loved.

Drunk

I have never been drunk in my life. I’ve never been buzzed or tipsy. The idea of losing the bit of control I have scares me. I fear I may become violent, very violent. There is so much anger, hurt, and rage that I don't know what would happen if I were to let my guard down. It's better to not know. I’ve lived the scenarios in my head through my mind and my people. It wasn’t pretty. At the time, it seemed so real, but now I know it wasn’t, but I don’t want to see real because I have no idea what real is. And I don’t want to know.

Alex & Harry

Alex and Harry are lovers. They exist, and they are perfect. No one dislikes them, no one distrusts them, no one disrespects them. Their love is perfect pure, and enduring. There s nothing they cannot deal with and overcome together. Their world is perfect and so far from mine. Yet, I feel as though I am connected to their world, and they are to mine. All that is good in my life is connected to theirs.

I know that they are a hallucination. I'm well aware of that fact . But they have been around so long they seem so real to me. Everything about them seems real. Because of them I knew what being gay meant long before my brothers learned about it. It just kind of filled in a space in my brain.

The Hulk man

The hulk man chases me, screaming. He jumps out, screaming at me when I least expect it. I never see him coming, and he scares me.

The first time I saw him, I just thought he was a man out for a run. Until he ran straight at me screaming. I fell over trying to get away and sobbed all the way back home.

I've not seen him on the road since, but he has come at me in the kitchen a few times, always screaming in my face knocking me down and always making my heart jump and race. He is a demon of the worst form.

The Photo Album

The photo album just made me angry. I had asked for years and years for my photos albums. There were two of them. I was constantly refused one or both.

When Patrick and Ann learned that I had seen the hospital files and comments they had made, I received a package in the mail. The box contained a third album with select photos inside.

Ann had specifically chosen posed photos where I was told to smile or were from my birthday parties and involved some elaborate cake. There were no sporting photos, no guiding photos, no choir or drama performance photos.

To add insult to injury, every birthday photo had different kids in the background. No one kid ever showed up in a second birthday photo. It was different kids each year. Truth be told, I only have contact with one of those kids now, and it's been that way for a very, very long time. It just goes to show that my childhood was a farce of false smiles and fake friends. I regret ever asking for those photos.

The early photos

The little girl in the photos shows just how bad things were. There are no false pretenses or poses n those early photos. The child is confused, sullen and looks scared. It pretty much sums up my early life. They are the only “baby” photos I have. Given to social workers for my file. I feel bad for that little girl. I wish I could give her a hug and tell her it's going to be okay. It really only ever was okay. It should have been wonderful. They had the means and had the money and resources to make it wonderful and didn’t.

The Glass Hospital

I once found myself in the strangest hospital I had ever encountered. It reminded me of jail with a common glassed-in area with glassed-in rooms encircling the common area. On the far side sat the staff watching and listening to everything said and done among the patients.

I had arrived the night before against my will after being transferred from the local hospital. I had fought tooth and nail against the transfer to the point where I had even cracked my head against the concrete.

I remember that part vividly. I remember the woman with me whispering to the hospital receptionist and being whisked back to a back room where a doctor insisted on knowing what my plans were. I had none; I just felt rotten. I felt lost, emotionless, and caught in the void, but I had no intention of telling them that. I had no intention of sharing anything. I refused to speak to them. So, they transferred me.

I spent a month in the new hospital begin stared at like a lion pacing behind the glass. The more they stared, the more agitated I got. The more agitated I got, the more they drugged me.

I spent a lot of my time drugged. I'd get agitated, they would drug me, I'd get agitated again, they would drug me again.

Pace, argue, sleep, pace, argue sleep. It was one hell of a month, and it did absolutely no good. By the time I got out, I felt worse than before. By that time, I had visions of running my car off the road and a powerful urge to do it.

No, I didn't do it. I didn't even try it. I had a child to care for. I just suffered in silence. Every day feeling worse and worse. Nightmares, visions, shadow people and the never-ending feeling of hopeless despair. The medication they gave me was supposed to help, but it didn't. So, I just forced myself to carry on as best as I could.

Whenever I could, I would withdraw to the scenarios in my head and the perfect world I could make for myself when my demons were quiet, and my people were gone. If the hum was low and I could work around it, I would spend hours each day in my own universe ignoring everything around me. If my people were there, I'd talk to them instead. If my demons were loud, I'd take extra meds and try to sleep them away—that only worked for so long. My pharmacist caught on to my early and frequent refills. Losing my meds was an excuse that only worked so often. I considered alcohol or other meds, but I didn't want to be incoherent or drunk; I just wanted to sleep and escape what was in my head.

Did I or Didn’t I

Did I or didn’t I. I spend a lot of time asking myself this question. Did I really do that, or was it someone else? Did I see it on tv, read it in a book, or was it my people, demons, or imagination? There are so many scenarios in my head that are questionable that I dare not mention because I don’t know if they are real or not. Sometimes it tortures me to think that the life I think I’ve had is not really my life or things I think I didn’t do I really did. I call up the snapshots in my mind; those things I know are real. But it gets harder and harder to know the difference as time goes on. Am I the person I think I am? I feel so alien in my body. Like it's someone else’s, and these stores are theirs. That these accomplishments are theirs, and I have nothing to show for myself after all these years. Who am I? I don't know.

Hotel Dieu, God’s Hospital

I often think about the hospital and picture myself there. Oddly enough, it's calming, which is strange because I hate hospitals. Everything about them creeps me out. I spent a lot of time in hospitals as a kid, and nothing about them was calming or comforting to me. I spent plenty of time in them as an adult, and it didn't get any better with age. In my last hospital visit, I stayed 3 weeks in the psych ward. I got into two altercations with staff and, at one point, was convinced I had to remain perfectly still so the bald man in the room wouldn't steal my hair.

At one point, I actually started pulling it out to give it to him so he would leave me alone. At the time, it was so real I begged the staff to restrain me so I wouldn't move and he'd leave me alone. They obliged but then took the restraints off when they thought I was sleeping. I was horrified. So why do I find daydreaming about the psych ward a calming thing when I'm terrified of going back there? Who knows? Maybe because I have control in my thoughts which I don't have at the actual hospital. Maybe because deep down, as much as I hate the hospital, I know it's a safe place. Which it pains me to say like the basement of the theatre or the clearing in the woods. No one judges you there because everyone is there is concerned with their own issues. Either way, I spent hours walking through those halls in my head. Something I wish would stop, but it never does.

Screaming

When the screaming starts, my anxiety shoots through the roof. I spend my time and efforts trying to stay calm and not outwardly show what is happening in my head. If I am home alone, I melt to the floor, covering my head and crying until it stops. If I am not alone, I try to hide, usually in the bathroom or outside. I grit my teeth and sing nursery rhymes. The rhythm soothes. The repetitiveness helps, but the screaming is usually random. It starts unexpectantly and ends unexpectantly. It sounds like someone is dying, blood curtly screams. High pitched and awful.

I've broken many things, having dropped them suddenly when startled by the screaming. It's worse when the hum is present, and demons and people are talking. The noise can be so intense my head feels as it will explode. The screaming is horrendous.

The Institution

I have often wondered what it would be like to be institutionalized. I don't even know if such places still exist, but what must they be like in this day and age. I imagine they wouldn't be much different than a long-term stay in the psych ward. A hospital stay means things are bad. But it also means a break. Not just from reality but from responsibilities as well. The only voices demanding my time and attention would be the ones in my head. My demons and my people. No demands from the house, the job, the pets, or the family. While it does get lonely after a while, the first little while is so much quieter, even if my head is yelling.

There is only the pressure of the voices, and I'm protected from their harm in hospital. At home, they rage the children demand the animals demand the house demands and my husband eyes me every day gauging my level of functioning. I'm used to the scrutiny, but some days I yearn for quiet calm control to not have to give anything a second thought. I'm not entirely sure institutions were altogether bad in that regard.

Suicide

I don't belong in this world. I know this. I've known it for a very long time. Since I was very, very young, I have now that there was something different about me. I knew it wasn't good. I saw how people looked at me and noticed when I was treated differently than others. I noticed the bullying the unspoken annoyance at helping me or having anything to do with me. I remember a girl guide ceremony where the patrol leader had to bring me to present my next-level award before the troop leaders.

She grabbed my sleeve with a disgusted sigh and literally hauled me up to the front. Everyone noticed. How could they not? Yet no one said or did anything about her behaviour or attitude toward me. It was typical of my interactions with others. No one wanted anything to do with me, and I couldn't figure out why. I only knew that I didn't belong anywhere or with anyone; everyone was so against me that it was painful. As a small child, I thought about running away but had nowhere to go. Doreen had long since moved, and for whatever reason, she paid much less attention to me when she did visit.

As I got older, suicide was a constant thought crossing my mind. I was so lonely, unhappy, and unwanted. No matter the group, the class, or the activity, I stood alone. It was painfully obvious. I once found a medical excuse to get out of practice for the cross-country team in high school. It was a horrible day for me, and I couldn't deal with the taunts from some team members and the silent treatment from others. Several days later, we had a meet in another city. I was excited to go and felt good about the race until I hit the finish line. I was one of four girls running that race, and while I didn’t finish last in the race, I did finish last for my team.

When I got to the finish line, no one was there. I couldn’t understand as it was team protocol to cheer on every racer until the finish. We had already done it for the boys on the team. I had cheered until I was hoarse. But no one from my team wasn't at the finish line, not even my coach. They were nowhere to be seen.

I sat down and waited. NO one came. When I finally found the school van, they had all packed up and were pulling out when they spotted me. My coach's excuse was I was so quiet he almost forgot I was there. In reality, I wasn't there. I had waited at the finish line like I was instructed to do.

Heading home, I was so distraught that they had forgotten me and almost left without me. I had a major panic attack. My coach freaked and dropped me at the hospital before leaving and heading back home with the other students. Patrick had to come two hours drive to get me, and he was less than impressed. He didn't want to know what had happened. He wanted me to sit through the ride home quietly. I was so upset I didn't bother to protest. I seriously considered ending my life when I got home. I was so tired and so upset I couldn't do it. My demons screamed at me that I was useless, worthless, and a waste of space. I believed them.

The following Monday in Cross country, we watched the video for the finish line. After Nancy crossed the finish line, my coach said on the video, “that’s everyone,” and stopped recording. When I turned to look at him, he would not look at me. He had genuinely forgotten about me, and no one else on the team had cared.

I honestly should not have been surprised it was the story of my life. I was constantly forgotten, overlooked, or otherwise treated as a nuisance. Patrick always forgot me at Guides. I walked home in the dark from across town on many cold winter nights. I wandered off into the woods for hours at a time, and no one noticed. I ran off to do whatever my heart desired and, no one questioned where I was or what I was doing because they either forgot about me or were genuinely happy I wasn’t around.

If they only knew where I was or what I was thinking. Maybe they did care or wouldn't have cared. But I spent a lot of time climbing bridges, standing on overpasses, hiding in the woods and letting boys have their way. I honestly didn't care what happened to me at that point because I knew no one else did. I came so close so many times. I didn't do it because I figured maybe just maybe someone might miss me. Also, I was scared. My demons told me I'd go to hell. The church said I'd go to hell. Patrick and Ann said I'd go to hell. I was scared of hell. What I realized was I was already in hell; I just didn't know it. Everyone hated me. I didn't belong, and I was stuck between the real world and some strange place that constantly occupied my thoughts. I was haunted by strange people and tormented by demons, and I was only 15 years old.

In my shoes

I have always wondered what other people would do in my shoes. What they would have done all those years ago. Would they have done the things I did, like eating the comet cleanser under the sink after being told it was poison?

Would they have stayed on the bridge, or would they have jumped? Would they have told someone about the pills or just slinked off somewhere quietly? I often wonder why I'm still here. What it is that stops me from doing it. I've come so close so many times, but I always stop. Is it fear? Is it God? I don't know. One day I will probably do it. But it won't matter because likely no one will notice.

No Happy Endings

I used to think that someday my real parents would come back for me. That they were wonderful people who just needed time to get it all straight. I didn't want to believe my mother was ill or disturbed or couldn't care for me. I didn't want to think I was so unloved that no one had wanted me. But they never came looking. They never came back for me. So, I accepted that I wasn't a missing princess or Annie or even Anne of Green Gables, who all found amazing families in the end.

I was the kid no one wanted. No one wanted to love me, no one wanted to be friends with me, and no one wanted to give me a chance.

I was just the weird kid that was given away. There are no happy endings. But I endure.

Truth be told there is so much more to the story and believe it or not there finally is justice for Jenny

Jenny Part 2 available December 2021

www.ingramcontent.com/pod-product-compliance
Ingram Content Group UK Ltd.
Pitfield, Milton Keynes, MK11 3LW, UK
UKHW020416250726
13967UKWH00007B/2679